LIMITLESS HEALTH

BY LAUREN DENOS

TABLE OF CONTENTS

LIVE YOUR LIFE WITHOUT LIMITS!

This workbook goes over 13 steps to help you identify your overall goals and then create the health goals that correlate to the life you would like to live. It also helps you with all the motivation and details that go along with goal setting. In this workbook you will learn to identify obstacles and find solutions so that nothing will stop you.

Use these tools to help you achieve the health you want for the life you desire and...

LIVE FULL OUT!

A HUGE THANK YOU!

I am very blessed to have a lot of amazing, talented, and supportive people in my life. So I would like to give a quick shout out to a few of these people.

Thank you to my artist team! The cover artwork is an awesome combination effort of Regina Rollis (Concept art), Sophia Diaz (Graphic arts), and Criss Madd (Character artwork). You all are amazingly talented artists that really put a lot of time, thought, and care into this cover. Thank you!

I have been very honest with people that I was not planning on being a writer, However as life would have it, that's what happened - I am someone who has experience in a field and I want to share this knowledge, and writing seemed like a good way. It is finally sinking in that I'm now a writer, but my grammar still gets the magical touch from Rachel Christine. Thank you for your editing so that I look literate!

My parents have always encouraged me to follow my own path and to do what I want with my life. That is the reason this workbook, and every other book I have written or ever will write is being created. Thank you mom and dad for telling me to do what I love.

My husband, Arthur, is the most amazing person in the world. He understands my need for adventure and exploration. He believes in what I do, deals with my obsessive work habits, my wild whims and supports me through it all. It takes a special man to do that. Thank you! I love you more than words can convey.

Thank you to all the people who have read this workbook while in progress and who gave me feedback to make sure that it's excellent for everyone else. Thank you to all of the people who surround me and make what I do possible and worthwhile, you rock!

WHY IS GOAL SETTING IMPORTANT TO YOUR LIFE?

"Setting goals is the first step in turning the invisible into the visible"
~ Tony Robbins

I would venture to say that nothing can change your life quite the way that goal setting can. Think about it, if you have no idea where you want to go how the heck do you know where to steer your life? Test this out. Right now, I want you to start doing jumping jacks, if you cannot do jumping jacks think of an exercise you can do right now where you are at. Okay set this book down and go do that exercise.

How did you do? How many did you do? Could you have done more? How long did it take? Did you pay attention to any of that information? This is how many people approach their lives. No goal, no plan, and no idea where they are going, or even where they want to be. If you take the time to map out your goals and pay attention to what you are doing, you can accomplish so much more. If you did 90 jumping jacks just a moment ago and you had set a goal before hand of 100 jumping jacks, do you think you would have pushed yourself to do those last ten? Probably. You can see how having these goals set ahead of time can make you more productive.

Why are we setting goals? Because if you do not give yourself a road map then you have no idea what direction you would like to go in. If you have no destination that is exactly where you will go, to a random somewhere or nowhere. Too many people leave their future up to chance. I do believe in fate and destiny and all of that, but at the same time we must give it a hand. You may have a possible destiny, but if you do nothing towards it to help that destiny along then it may not happen. Taking action and destiny go hand in hand. For instance, if you are being given opportunities or having thoughts toward being a painter and you keep ignoring it, or you keep saying "yeah someday," you are not putting in the action towards your destiny. Therefore your chances of anything happening towards it are very slim to none.

I have done this in the past. I was too scared to do what I needed to do, and let's just say the results were very bad. Through this, I have come to realize that I need to pay attention to the ideas and instincts I have, and do my part to see them to fruition. Does that mean I accomplish all of them right away? No. Rather, it means I acknowledge them and then decide what the right order is for these goals. While some goals are meant to be jumped on right away, others are meant to be thought on and built upon.

Have you ever met someone who was upset with life because they wanted more, but when you ask them what they would like in their life, they couldn't tell you?

A good example of this is my friend Becky. She did not like what she was doing with her life, and wanted more. The problem was, she didn't know what she wanted. Because of this she had been in a rut for a while. Becky is very sweet woman with a lot of potential, but she just had not put much thought into what she wanted. I helped her to create a goal chart and a vision board, a vision board is a collection of pictures usually put on a poster board that represent what you would like to accomplish, it is like a goal list but with pictures.

Once she started to think about what she wanted and put them into words, her life started changing. She left the low-income, dead-end job she was in and went to school. She graduated school and is now working in career she loves. She told me that almost everything on her vision board has been accomplished! In fact, seeing her goals every day helped her know where she was headed and kept her moving in the right direction.

If you have no goals, then how do you know where you want to go? I don't know about you, but I don't want to leave my life up to chance like that!

I have another friend, Jessica, who kept making New Year's resolutions and other health goals throughout the year. They would only generally last a month, maybe three if she was really using her willpower. Eventually, though, her efforts would always fizzle out. I talked to her about her goals, and she would always have these goals of being a certain weight or fitting into a size 6. But when I asked her why she wanted to accomplish this, she could not tell me. In that moment, she discovered what the issue was. It is not that she could not lose the weight, it was that she did not set the proper goals for it. Having goals that mean something to you gives you an ultimate reason of why you are doing something. As we probed what was important to her, we discovered that her family was a big deal. She wanted to be a good role model for her kids. In order to do that, she needed to be healthy so she could go do activities with her family. Once this was figured out and she finally knew what her true goals were, we had something more to work with and it made planning a lot easier. She planned her fitness routines, nutrition, and cooked healthy meals with her new family-oriented goals in mind. In addition, she created exercises the whole family could do together. Eventually, she achieved a leaner body and met her more important goals that had to do with her family. She is now able to keep her fitness and health where she wants it and knows where she is going with her health.

Be honest about what you want with your life. Having an altruistic goal is fine if it is really what you want, but if you are making a life goal of helping the world and feeding the hungry but what you really want is to travel the world and be a world class speaker, then you are not going to be using the right motivations for yourself. Remember when you focus on what you really want in life, you will be more motivated to accomplish the health you want as well. This does not mean you will not do the altruistic things you want as well, it just may not be as powerful of a motivational point. Let's get started!

STEP 1 – WHAT KIND OF LIFE DO YOU WANT?

"Life isn't about finding yourself. Life is about creating yourself"
~ *George Brenard Shaw*

In this step we will talk about how to find your overall goal. First look at where are you at in your life? Are you happy with your life how it is? Do you feel like you could use a change? If a change is what you seek then start with what you are doing with your life, also look at your work, after all, our "work" is a big majority of our lives. If you love what you are doing already then that is great! You are one step closer to identifying what kind of health you should focus on to maximize your life, if not, then let's find out what you want.

What do you see as your ultimate life? I personally believe that many of us have a certain passion, and that is what we are meant to do with our lives. Do you have something that you really love?

When you think about what you love to do, don't not worry about what's realistic. I ask people, "if you could do anything with your life, no limitations, what would you do?" At first many people say, "hmm, I think I would like to be an accountant." Okay, for some maybe that really is their dream, but many people who are answering that way, are really just thinking - "What can I make money at and not hate." When you are asked this question, think about what you really love to do. That thing that you would spend all your free time doing –fishing, dancing, skydiving, playing video games etc. You can make a living out of just about anything, all you need is a little creative thinking.

First you have to find out what you love to do, then you can start getting creative on how you could make money from it. Write down all the ideas that come into your head no matter how stupid they might seem. Keep writing until you can't think of anything else, and then think a little more. The craziest trains of thought may yield an idea you never thought of before.

You can do this exercise alone or get a friend or a group of friends to brain storm with you. You would be amazed at what can be accomplished when you have a group of minds together to throw ideas around. Again do not worry about being realistic when you do your brain storming, just let it flow.

Think about this. If you love fishing, you could easily be a fishing guide, or you could own a fishing guide company. What's more, you could create a fishing magazine, do a TV show on fishing, or you could even open a fishing supply shop! These were just a few ideas off the top of my head. The point is you can think of ways to make money at anything! This does not mean that you should give up your current job right away. It just means that you can start making plans to get to the ultimate job of your dreams.

Find some quiet time to really think about what you would like to have in your life. Jot down ideas as they come into your head. This is good to do on a regular basis since so many people have so many things they would like to do with their life. Sometimes, it can get overwhelming and you can get distracted and pulled in different directions, ultimately accomplishing nothing. Sit down with a notepad in case you need more room than what is provided in this workbook, write down all the things you would like to do. This can help clarify a lot. When you do this imagine yourself doing the work for the goal you are wanting to accomplish and see yourself completing this goal, this will serve as a mental rehearsal to show you if this is something you would really like to spend your time on. For me some of my goals are ones that will be put to the forefront as most important to accomplish now, and some of them will go on the back burner and I can be working on the skills for them so that I can accomplish them down the road. No matter how "unrealistic" your goal may be, write it down on this list and think of why you want it. No matter how big your goal is you can accomplish it, especially when you create a plan of action.

* If you cannot think of a big overall life goal, do not worry. Instead you can think of something in the moment you would like to achieve. This is a way to get the ball rolling, and will all develop and change in your life. So if you do not have an overall life goal thought up, do not stress about it. Just think of what you would currently like to achieve. Whether it's being better at your job, being able to move easier, to get through your day without being exhausted, or just being able to play with your kids, it is a great place to start. It will progress naturally from there.

Here is an example of a list of overall life goals: (yours may be different.)

Example list
To be a....
Public Speaker
Author
Expert in my field
Top sales person
Adventurer
Actor
Writer for a column in a magazine

Or to...
Create a clothing line
Start your own company (be specific on the type of company)
Start a wilderness program for troubled youth
....The possibilities are endless

<u>Start your list of all the things you might want to do here.</u>

_____
_____
_____
_____
_____
_____
_____
_____
_____
_____
_____
_____
_____
_____

Go back through the list you just made and do a mental rehearsal of each of these overall goal ideas. Make sure when you do the rehearsal that you visualize all the hard parts of it too, not just the awesome parts. You may think having a business of your own is great until you start to look at all the detailed, tedious work that goes into it. You want to make sure you think it through, so that you better understand what you really want. After you do a mental rehearsal of each one put a star next to the ones you think you would enjoy the most.

Look at these and number them from the ones you would like to do most at this time to the ones you might like to look at doing down the road.

So what do you want to do with your life? What is your overall life goal? Pick the top one you would like to work on:

_____
_____
_____
_____
_____

Create a detailed image of what it will look like when you accomplish this goal. What does it look like?

_____
_____
_____
_____
_____

How do you feel when you see yourself accomplishing this goal?

_____

_____

_____

_____

_____

_____

_____

_____

_____

_____

If applicable: How can you make a living doing this?

_____

_____

_____

_____

_____

_____

_____

_____

_____

STEP 2- WHO, WHAT, WHY AND LOOK INSIDE!

"When we lose the right to be different, we lose the privilege to be free"
~ Charles Evans Hughes

Look at what you want and why you want it. Make sure that you are setting goals for the right reasons. Make sure they are for you, not some mold you are wanting to fit into because of what society, your parents or friends tell you that you should be.

- What do you want?

- Why do you want it?

- How will this change your life?

- Why have you not done this before?

- Where did this goal come from?

- Is this what you want or what others have pushed onto you?

The answers to these questions are important because they tell you if the person you are working towards being is who you really want to be, or if you are working towards fitting a mold that you haven't chosen for yourself.

If you find that you are working towards fitting a mold that you haven't chosen for yourself you are more likely to get off track.

For example:
Let's say one of your overall goals is to be in the top 10% in your industry. Is this goal from you really loving your industry? Did it come from the need to feel accomplished? If so is this the area you really want to focus on being successful in? Is it because your parents expect you to be the best in this industry? Is this something you decided on a whim or have you really thought this through over some time? Remember, your goal needs to be something YOU want. If you are doing this for someone other than you, it is harder to really succeed in your goal to the level that you are hoping for.

I knew a guy who went to medical school and specialized in anesthesiology. Medical school, as we all know, is a long (10 year) process, and it is worth it if it is what you would like to do. This man in particular was doing this because it is what was expected of him, and I am sure for some of the prestige. He got all the way through school and was practicing medicine, I saw him one day and asked him how he was enjoying his new career, and he told me he hated it! So, I asked him what he is going to do instead. His response was he was going to be an anesthesiologist! Here is a man that hates what he is doing, but is going to keep doing it because of what is expected of him.

Would you want to live a life where you hate what you do? How would you feel if you were going to see a doctor that hated what they do? I would not want to see them. If someone hates what they do they are most likely not going to be up to speed on the current issues in their industry, and therefore will not be giving you the best service. I would rather go to someone who loves what they do. When someone loves what they do, they are one of the best! You know they are studying it every chance they get because they really enjoy it.

Many times we say we want something, but it is not really what we want but what we think we *should* want. Make sure when you are setting goals that they are for you. This process helps to dig into why you really want this goal, or if it is really what you want at all. These can be looked at all the time to remind yourself of why you are working on this goal. Keep adding to this list if you think of something else later on.

I know too many women who aim to look like fitness models even though this has nothing to do with what they really want. It seems to be one of the more common goals in our society. Don't get me wrong, there is nothing wrong with a goal like this. The problem, however, is if it is not what you really want you have a higher chance of not achieving it and then feeling like a loser because of not succeeding. If this is the case, you are not a loser, it is just not what you really want. You may wind up having a super fit body from focusing on what you want, but it is not your main goal. Let's say what you really want is to hike the Himalayas, you very well could get into fitness model shape by training for this, but the fitness model body is not your focus. The hike is what motivates you.

Many people have no idea what they would like to do with their lives. Usually this is because they have not been paying attention to the signs along the way. Is there a passion that you have? Something that has been on your mind or something you are naturally good at? I believe that our passion in life is our mission on this planet. So listen to your passions. It is important that you are being honest with what you want with your life, and not what someone else is telling you to do.

Time to answer the questions we talked about above. It is important that we write things down, otherwise they may stay just a thought with no action or movement behind them. Fill in the answers to the questions on the next page.

What do you want?

_____

_____

_____

_____

Why do you want it?

_____

_____

_____

_____

How will this change your life?

_____

_____

_____

_____

Why have you not done this before?

_____

_____

_____

_____

Where did this goal come from?

_____

_____

_____

_____

Is this what you want or what others have pushed on you?

_____

_____

_____

_____

STEP 3- GET IN SHAPE FOR YOUR IDEAL LIFE

" Health is the soul that animates all enjoyments of life, which fade and are tasteless without it" ~ Lucius Annaeus Seneca

Your overall goals will lead to your health goals and your health directly affects what you are able to accomplish in your daily life. Are you really accomplishing all you would like to? What kind of health do you need to develop for the specific life goals you have?

What is your life goal? This will be your guiding star to your fitness and nutrition goals. If your main goal in life is to be at the top of your business field, then you may not have the time to workout a few times a day. If your goal is to be a top rated endurance hiker, then eating a full balanced meal every 2 or 3 hours may not fit with your goal.

Many people, when they think about their health and fitness, think that they need to look like a fitness model and that becomes their goal. Yet that is not what they actually want, and therefore fail over and over again until they get so frustrated they stop attempting to get healthy at all. Can you see how if your real goal in life is to have the #1 bestselling book why the fitness model goal may not work for you? Because you are using the wrong motivation for yourself. If you want to be a #1 bestselling author, think of how working out would give you better mental clarity and better stamina to write and deal with book tours. Thinking this way, you just may get into a fitness model shape while you are working towards your goal, but you are using a motivation that works for you. Plus if you do not get into fitness model shape it is not stressing you out because it is not your main focus. Being honest with yourself will take you far.

There is no wrong goal for you to choose. However, it must be what YOU want, not what society says you should want. The easiest way to get healthy is to get real with yourself about what is important to you and what you want from life.

Some examples are:
• To excel in my career
• To have a close family life
• To be financially secure
• To be an adventurer

The possibilities are endless. There is no right or wrong when it comes to what you want. Once you have a general idea of your goal, you can start to make it more detailed.

For Instance

If your goal in life is to excel in your career. What type of career is it? What kind of health do you need to have to be even better at it? It may be that you simply need to have a sharper, clearer mind. Or maybe you need to travel a lot and therefore you want your body to be able to handle all the jet lag better. Maybe your job needs you to look a certain way to be an example for clients. You may be able to get in a meal every 3-4 hours or you may be only able to get three meals in a day.

If you would like to have a closer family, then maybe you want to be a good example for your children so that they grow up healthy. Maybe you would like to have the energy to play with your children. If you have illness that runs in the family, then maybe you are fighting against that so that you can stay around longer for your children.

If one of your goals is to be financially secure, then maybe what you are looking for is good health to deal with the demanding hours you are working, cultivating a sharp mind to see opportunities when they come your way. Your nutrition and fitness would focus on this criteria.

If your goal is to be an adventurer, what types of adventures do you want to go on? Do you need tons of strength and stamina for your adventures? You probably need energy. You may realistically only have time to eat 3 solid meals and maybe snacks on the trails. So your eating plan would need to reflect that.

The point here is to tailor what you are doing with your health and fitness to what you want to accomplish in life. Once you know what you want out of life, you can decide what type of body and health you will need to get there. Health can mean so many different things. You have to choose what health means to you.

You may have many goals rather than one goal you would like to focus on in your life, and that is great, it just means that you will have a multifaceted plan. So if you want to run some marathons for the fun of it but for your career you build sculptures out of heavy materials you would need to have a combination of cardio training, core strength, and weight training for all the heavy lifting you do.

Look at what type of health you think you would need to have for your main life goal. The fitness plan that a figure competitor would follow verses a mom wanting to stay active so she can keep up with her kids, is going to be very different.

Example #1

Let's take an example of a man who is a computer tech. We will call him Frank. Now, Frank loves his career, but has some back pain due to his posture at work. He wants to get rid of the back pain and have more energy throughout the day. He also would like to start taking vacations in the mountains to do some hiking.

First of all, what will give him energy? Is he getting 8 hours of sleep? If not, that will be one of the first suggestions. The body does most of its repairing while we sleep, so if he is not getting enough sleep it would make sense that the body is not feeling it's best.

Next step is with eating, is he eating often enough? What type of food is he eating? He would want to make sure he is getting a meal in at least 3 times a day. Four to six small meals a day would be great to keep energy up, but it depends on what he has already been doing, what kind of time he has available, and what his body needs. I would be happy with him at least getting three meals in a day. What's more, I would suggest he have some protein, vegetables, carbohydrates, and fats at each meal, as well as some healthy carbs such as quinoa, sweet potatoes or whole grains. Though, this all depends on his specific body and his habits. There is, of course, an ideal way for us to eat for our bodies, but we must also be realistic on what people are willing to do.

For instance, let's say to be healthy Frank has to give up all of his favorite food. He would most likely not stick with this new way of eating. In order to work effectively, his plan needs to be realistic. The nutrition changes wouldn't happen otherwise. If Frank eats fast food every day and really likes it, then cuts out the fast food entirely, this would be a recipe for failure. Instead, he would do better to determine some healthier alternatives and go from there. Something Frank could start doing is making at least one meal a day at home. Nutrition is one of the most important aspects of our health. As they say, abs are made in the kitchen, this means the basis of your health is what you put in your body.

Following this example, we want to change things gradually. If we change our routine all at once, we will more than likely rebel. But, if we change things slowly we are more likely to stick with it, we would then see the good changes taking place.

After that is squared away, Frank should start a weight training routine that would cover the whole body, and pay special attention to his back and legs. He may also want to throw in a bit of stretching or yoga for his back as well. Next for his hiking goal he needs to get a bit more walking in, focusing on hilly areas in particular. On the weekends, he should hit some good hiking trails so he is prepared for the big vacation trails. There are many more suggestions for this like: having proper shoes and support, working in a chair that is supportive for his back, sitting up straight. You get the picture here. We now have a great idea of the health goals he would make to support his overall goals.

Example #2

Let's look at an example from the other end of the spectrum. Jennifer wants to be in the Olympics, she's going for the hurdles. She is definitely going to need that full 8 hours of sleep. In fact, it will be vital that she gets a good night's rest every night. She will be training so intensely that she needs to let her body repair. In addition, her diet would be much more precise. Vegetables and lean healthy meats will be important, as well as a good amount of healthy carbohydrates and fats. She will need to have them in the right proportions depending on her body, she will be needing way more calories than the average person. Jennifer will also most likely need some supplements to help her system recover. Training and eating will be broken down into a precise schedule.

Jennifer's training regimen would be pretty grueling. It may be comprised of distance running, plyometrics, and weight training focused on the lower body and core muscles. Her goal list would be focused on her times for runs as well as on her jumps and precise eating.

Let's look at some other examples:

If you are really ambitious and you have a whole handful of goals like having a great business, becoming an international public speaker, Author and Adventurer.

What kind of health would you need to accomplish all of this? Just a few things you may need are:

- Need to have a clear head which means, eat foods that promote that. (for you it could mean free of grains or sugars or dairy or all of them).
- Need to look healthy for your speaking, this means hitting the gym and doing weight training as well as eating for a healthy body.
- Need to have amazing stamina and strength for any adventures you choose to go on..

Let's say your goal is to be the best, attentive mother and the best role model possible. What you may need to accomplish this is:

- Keeping your energy up by doing regular exercise and eating right.
- Finding exercises that the whole family can do together.
- Creating healthy meals that the family will enjoy and letting your children help prepare the meals.
- Healthy sleeping habits for the whole family.

What if your overall goal is to be the best (Motorcycle) racer in the world? What you may want to do to get there is:

- Create more stamina by working on your cardiovascular abilities.
- Better core stability. Your core strength is super important while riding and turning at high speed.
- Eat for clarity, alertness and leanness. Let's face it, if you are riding and making split decisions at that speed, you need to be super alert and clear about what you are doing, and the lighter you are the faster you will be.
- Strength training so that you can handle the bike better.

Can you see how much stronger the motivation can be when it is something you are really wanting in life? Knowing what you want is the first step, yet so many people ignore this important step. So here is your chance to start with what is really important to you.

What is your overall goal? (This will be what you discovered in the previous chapters)

_____
_____
_____
_____
_____
_____

What kind of health goals do you need to succeed in this overall goal?

_____
_____
_____
_____
_____
_____
_____
_____
_____
_____
_____
_____
_____
_____
_____

STEP 4 - TURNING GOALS INTO ACTION STEPS!

"When it is obvious that the goals cannot be reached, don't adjust the goals, adjust the action steps"~ Confucius

In the last step we talked about what kind of health you need to have so you can achieve what you want in your life. Now let's take this a step further. Now we will go over all the smaller goals and action steps that you will create to accomplish the goals that you have set. Once you know what your overall goals are, you can decide what you need to do to support these goals. So if your overall goal is to be in the top 10% of your industry. You have determined that in order to be the best you should have better mental clarity, stamina, and look aesthetically pleasing to deal with clients. Now you will look at what health and fitness action steps you would need to set to accomplish that type of health. Let's look at what kind of action steps you would need to take. For instance to accomplish the better stamina, clarity, or better appearance we talked about previously. For clarity you may need to eat better foods that do not fog up the brain and get rid of the ones that do, like sugar or for some people it is grains or caffeine. Regarding your better body image, you may need to do some weight training. For stamina, add in some cardio. Let's look at some other examples of how this would look. Once you know what you need to do you will take these action steps and create smaller bite sized goals.

Example #1

If your overall goal is: To excel in your career as a sale woman and to raise a healthy family

In this case, you know that you are going to need to have a good amount of energy and stamina to keep up with two priorities that are this important, and can both take up quite a bit of your time and attention. You are going to have to think on your feet for your work. The benefits of what you are doing with your health and fitness is that you also become a good role model so that your kids will learn how to take care of themselves.

What you need	**Actions to accomplish it**
Better Stamina to keep up with your kids and work	Cardio weekly
Mental Clarity	Eliminate sugar and allergens
Energy	Get my sleep, eat as above, supplements

General goals created from my actions listed above
- 30 minutes of moderate cardio 3X a week, you can do this with your kids!
- Plan my meals out in advance.
- Replace all the highly refined carbs and sugary foods in my house with better alternatives.
- Create a schedule so that I get to bed on time.

Example #2
If your overall goal is: To be an actress

For a goal like this, you will need to be at the top of your game. You need to look good and be healthy, as well as having enough energy to keep up with the random auditions, shoots and a regular job. In everyday terms, this means good nutrition and exercise. You need to be able to adapt to whatever role you wind up landing, which means switching up your exercises regularly to keep your body versatile. If you are interested in action roles then you need to take your level of fitness to a whole different level, you would probably then want to take up boxing or martial arts classes.

What you need	**Actions to accomplish it**
Energy to keep up with a job and auditions	Get enough sleep, have a healthy diet
A healthy physique	A healthy diet, a variety of exercise
Adaptability	Having a wide range of exercises

General goals created from my actions listed above
- 30 minutes of moderate to intense cardio 5X a week and weight training 3X a week.
- Plan my meals out in advance.
- Replace all the refined carbs and sugary foods in my house with better options.
- Make time for naps if schedule is not permitting a regular sleep schedule.

Example #3
If your overall goal is: To be a successful business owner

For this goal, you know you will most likely be working long hours. So you will either have to schedule in a block of time for your exercises or find short times throughout the day for mini workouts. You may want something as simple as walks to reduce stress and keep your blood oxygenated so you can keep up your energy and focus. Nutrition will be a big key factor for you since it is the best way to keep your body healthy and your mind sharp.

What you need	**Actions to accomplish it**
Mental clarity	Healthy diet full of veggies
Energy	Healthy diet and exercise
Stress relief	Exercise and walking

General goals created from my actions listed above
- Short walks throughout every work day.
- Plan meals out and cut out the sugars and processed foods.
- For stress you may want to take up boxing or weight training 3X a week.

Be honest about what you want. If you lie about this, the only one you are hurting is yourself. This is for *your* motivation. So you can create a healthy lifestyle and make it stick!

Use the spaces below for what you have discovered in step 3 and 4.

What I need   Actions to accomplish it

_____   _____
_____   _____
_____   _____
_____   _____
_____   _____
_____   _____
_____   _____

General goals created from my actions listed above

_____
_____
_____
_____
_____
_____
_____
_____
_____
_____

STEP 5 – WHY DO YOU WANT TO ACCOMPLISH THIS GOAL?

"He who has a why to live can bear almost any how." ~*Friedrich Nietzsche*

So you have figured out your goal and you have figured out how you are going to make it happen. But you must also know the reasons you want to accomplish this goal. Knowing this will help you stick with it when obstacles get in the way and the going gets tough. When you fall of the band wagon your reasons for setting this goal will help bring you back onto the path.

A great way to do this, is to get a friend to ask you what is so important about accomplishing this goal. For this one let's take the example of wanting more energy. So your friend would ask, "What is so important about having better energy?" You would answer the first reason that pops into your head. Let's say your answer is "so I can be more productive". Then next they would ask "What is so important about being productive", and you may answer "So I can make more money". They will keep asking this many times. No less than around 20 times and they keep writing down the answers you give. You can continue this as long as you need to get to the heart of what you find important about your goal. Twenty times should be your minimum, but you can go longer. This gives you a frame work to understand what is important to you.

Example:

Q: What is so important to you about having more energy?
A: So that I can be more productive.
Q: What is so important to you about being more productive?
A: So that I can make better money.
Q: What is so important to you about making better money?
A: So that I can take better care of my family.
Q: What is so important to you about taking better care of your family?
A: So I can feel accomplished

When you have the right reasons behind your goal it is so much easier to stick with it. It motivates you. If you can not find motivation behind the goal you want then you may need to rethink what you are aiming for. Your reasons do not need to be normal or conventional and it does not matter if anyone else understands it. It is *your* reason for *your* goal and *your* life. Start to live it that way!

Let's look at your goal/goals. If you have multiple goals then do this exercise for each one. You may want a separate sheet of paper if you are doing multiple goals.

What is so important about ?_____

_____

What is so important about ?_____

_____

What is so important about ?_____

_____

What is so important about ?_____

_____

What is so important about ?_____

_____

What is so important about ?_____

_____

What is so important about ?_____

_____

What is so important about ?_____

_____

What is so important about ?_____

_____

What is so important about ?_____

_____

What is so important about ?_____

_____

What is so important about ?_____

_____

What is so important about ?_____

_____

What is so important about ?_____

_____

What is so important about ?_____

_____

What is so important about ?_____

_____

What is so important about ?_____

_____

What is so important about ?_____

_____

What is so important about ?_____

_____

Take these answers and write them on the lines below. Post these somewhere you will see them. This way you will be reminded of why you are working towards these goals.

My Goal is: _____

This goal is important because...

_____
_____
_____
_____
_____
_____
_____

My Goal is: _____

This goal is important because...

_____
_____
_____
_____
_____
_____
_____

My Goal is: _____

This goal is important because...

_____
_____
_____
_____
_____
_____
_____

STEP 6- GOAL CHARTING

"People with goals succeed because they know where they're going" ~ *Earl Nightingale*

In this chapter we will take a look at my favorite style of goal charting. There are many types of goal charts, but I feel this one gets more in-depth then others do. It does take longer to put together since I tend to do an entire year at once, but it is worth the effort. I love that I have everything laid out by the week so I know exactly what I need to do to stay on target for what I want to accomplish. I do find myself having to edit my goal chart a few times throughout the year. This is because I will create these charts with what is going on in my life at the moment in mind, but these things change. You may change jobs, decide that you would like to pursue something else. Anything can happen. But when I do the full years goal chart, I still have the frame work, I just edit it from there. This is a chart you can use for either just your fitness goals of for everything and anything. I personally chart out all of my goals on these charts. A good reason to lay out the whole year at once is because the goals you want to accomplish later in the year will have an impact on what you plan for this month. If you plan to have lost 10% body fat by the end of the year, then you need to be working on that this month. If you are planning on having a new job in three months, then the action steps you are taking towards that needs to be reflected in the months leading up to it. Let's start with some examples.

Example
- Run my first marathon
- Plan my food
- Do a fun activity with my family each weekend

You can do more than what I am showing in the upcoming examples. For now start with just one or only a few goals and then you can build it up from there if you want. You do not want to overload yourself by charting out 20 different goals

With this example we will look at how to place goals into a 12-month map. We will place these goals in a realistic time frame. For example when running a first marathon, if you have never done any running before now then you may want to plan that for 6 month to a year from now depending on your level of health. Let's say it is January right now and you decide to put the marathon goal in December. Then we want to look at cutting down the marathon goal into medium sized goals or steps. So we would put a 1/2 marathon in June and a 5k in April. Then you will look at what weekly marks you will need to hit to accomplish this goal. This is how you will work all of your goals. Look at what is a realistic time frame to accomplish them and then break it down. I have given examples of how all three items listed above would look in this layout.

Example: From the 3 health goals we were just looking at.

January: Start planning dinners throughout the week
Find one activity the family will enjoy together, do that every other weekend

February: Find a few more activities that the family will enjoy and plan something 3 weekend days

March: Plan Dinners and lunches through the week

April: Run a 5k
Find a few more activities that the family will enjoy and plan something 4 weekend days

May: Plan Dinners, Lunches and Breakfasts throughout the week

June: Run a half marathon

July:

August: Be prepping all but special night out meals.

September:

October:

November:

December: Run my first marathon.

Do you see how we put our big goals in the months we want to accomplish them, and then worked backwards? We would fill in the more distant months like December and then break them down.
Your turn. What are your fitness goals?

_____
_____
_____
_____
_____
_____
_____
_____

Next break these goals into mile stones just like we did on the previous page.

January:

February:

March:

April:

May:

June:

July:

August:

September:

October:

November:

December:

Now that you know what your milestone goals are you can look at what you need to do throughout the weeks to accomplish these goals. This is the meat and potatoes of this process. You can have big pie in the sky dreams; but, if you do not take regular steps towards them, then they will always just be something in the future. In the chart on the next page, I have used the same 3 examples. Obviously yours will be different. Only you know your schedule and what is realistic. If you are working crazy hours and are lucky to get enough sleep, then you may only be able to squeeze in10 minutes for weight training. It is better than nothing. Do what works for you. You will also notice that many of your weeks will look very similar and that is okay. If you have a marathon goal you know you will have running in your chart every week. Some of your other training and food goals will probably be either the same or pretty darn similar from week to week. And then you will have the few things that change more often.

JANUARY GOALS!

Run 3 miles
Have two family fun activity days
Prepare dinners

□Choose 5-7 healthy dinners that the family will like.
□Weight train   □Tuesday   □Thursday
□Find one activity the family would enjoy and plan 2 weekend days this month for it.
□Run 1-2 miles □Monday   □Wednesday   □Friday
□Prep dinners for the week. ie:Cook chicken ahead of time so I can just throw the rest together.

□Choose 5-7 healthy dinners that the family will like.
□Weight train   □Tuesday   □Thursday
□Run 1-2 miles □Monday   □Wednesday   □Friday
□Prep the dinners for the week.
□ Family fun day Saturday.

□Choose 5-7 healthy dinners that the family will like.
□Weight train   □Tuesday   □Thursday
□Run 2-3 miles □Monday   □Wednesday   □Friday
□Prep dinners for the week.

□Choose 5-7 healthy dinners that the family will like.
□Weight train   □Tuesday   □Thursday
□Run 2-3 miles □Monday   □Wednesday   □Friday
□Prep dinners for the week.
□ Family fun day Saturday.

Obviously yours will look different. You can do one goal for now if you want, or do multiples. Do you see the week to week repetition I talked about? It will slightly change as you progress in your goals. And you may have some big things that come up in some weeks, but usually there is quite a bit of repetition. You want to print this out and check off your goals as you accomplish them, that is why all the charts have been designed with check boxes.

Your turn!
I have provided a page for all 12 months so it is easier to chart out your upcoming year.

JANUARY GOALS!

_____
_____
_____
_____
_____

- ☐
- ☐
- ☐
- ☐
- ☐

- ☐
- ☐
- ☐
- ☐
- ☐

- ☐
- ☐
- ☐
- ☐
- ☐

- ☐
- ☐
- ☐
- ☐
- ☐

FEBRUARY GOALS!

_____
_____
_____
_____
_____

- ☐
- ☐
- ☐
- ☐
- ☐

- ☐
- ☐
- ☐
- ☐
- ☐

- ☐
- ☐
- ☐
- ☐
- ☐

- ☐
- ☐
- ☐
- ☐
- ☐

MARCH GOALS!

_____
_____
_____
_____
_____

- ☐
- ☐
- ☐
- ☐
- ☐

- ☐
- ☐
- ☐
- ☐
- ☐

- ☐
- ☐
- ☐
- ☐
- ☐

- ☐
- ☐
- ☐
- ☐
- ☐

APRIL GOALS!

_____
_____
_____
_____
_____

- ☐
- ☐
- ☐
- ☐
- ☐

- ☐
- ☐
- ☐
- ☐
- ☐

- ☐
- ☐
- ☐
- ☐
- ☐

- ☐
- ☐
- ☐
- ☐
- ☐

MAY GOALS!

_____
_____
_____
_____
_____

- ☐
- ☐
- ☐
- ☐
- ☐

- ☐
- ☐
- ☐
- ☐
- ☐

- ☐
- ☐
- ☐
- ☐
- ☐

- ☐
- ☐
- ☐
- ☐
- ☐

JUNE GOALS!

_____
_____
_____
_____
_____

- ☐
- ☐
- ☐
- ☐
- ☐

- ☐
- ☐
- ☐
- ☐
- ☐

- ☐
- ☐
- ☐
- ☐
- ☐

- ☐
- ☐
- ☐
- ☐
- ☐

JULY GOALS!

_____

_____

_____

_____

_____

- ☐
- ☐
- ☐
- ☐
- ☐

- ☐
- ☐
- ☐
- ☐
- ☐

- ☐
- ☐
- ☐
- ☐
- ☐

- ☐
- ☐
- ☐
- ☐
- ☐

AUGUST GOALS!

_____
_____
_____
_____
_____

- ☐
- ☐
- ☐
- ☐
- ☐

- ☐
- ☐
- ☐
- ☐
- ☐

- ☐
- ☐
- ☐
- ☐
- ☐

- ☐
- ☐
- ☐
- ☐
- ☐

SEPTEMBER GOALS!

_____
_____
_____
_____
_____

☐
☐
☐
☐
☐

☐
☐
☐
☐
☐

☐
☐
☐
☐
☐

☐
☐
☐
☐
☐

OCTOBER GOALS!

_____
_____
_____
_____
_____

☐
☐
☐
☐
☐

☐
☐
☐
☐
☐

☐
☐
☐
☐
☐

☐
☐
☐
☐
☐

NOVEMBER GOALS!

_____
_____
_____
_____
_____

☐
☐
☐
☐
☐

☐
☐
☐
☐
☐

☐
☐
☐
☐
☐

☐
☐
☐
☐
☐

DECEMBER GOALS!

_____
_____
_____
_____
_____

- [ ]
- [ ]
- [ ]
- [ ]
- [ ]

- [ ]
- [ ]
- [ ]
- [ ]
- [ ]

- [ ]
- [ ]
- [ ]
- [ ]
- [ ]

- [ ]
- [ ]
- [ ]
- [ ]
- [ ]

STEP 7– OBSTACLES AND SOLUTIONS

"A hero is an ordinary individual who finds the strength to persevere and endure in spite of overwhelming obstacles" ~ Christopher Reeve

Obstacles are challenges that get in your way when you are working towards achieving your goals. Contrary to popular belief, obstacles are actually a very good sign. First of all, obstacles help you grow. Think about it, anytime you have come across an obstacle, whether you chose to get around it or not, that is when you learned the most and grew as a person. You had to think harder, work harder and many times had to go through significant, emotional times. This is what grows you.

Another great thing about obstacles, is that they are a sign that you are absolutely moving forward. Obstacles do not get in your way when you are standing still. Just let that sink in. As an example: There are two superheros climbing up a building, and there is a ledge 10 stories above them that is very difficult to get up and over. One superhero gets tired so he decides to stop, while the second superhero keeps climbing. Which one is going to come across the ledge (the obstacle)? The one who is moving forward (or up in this case). So if you look at them in this way you realize that obstacles are a great sign that you are moving forward on your goal or in life. Obstacles will never look the same to you.

Once you realize you have come up to an obstacle or block you need to find a solution. You don't want to dwell on the problem, acknowledge it, throw a quick tantrum or cry if you need to and then move on to how you are going to work around it. Be a solution minded person. You will be amazed at how many obstacles become blessings when you focus on solutions. Often the biggest "problem" that comes up turns out to be the best thing that could have happened. It was your catalyst for change.

Example # 1
What if you are doing a computer desk job where you type all day, and you break your wrist? Your boss decides that he cannot wait for you to heal and fires you. This, at first, would seem like the worst thing that could possibly happen. However, since you are a solution finder you decide to make a list of all the options to get around this obstacle. You decide to put a few options on your list (you are about to create) into effect and wind up finding a job that is better than anything you could have imagined. You would have never found this new great job had this obstacle not occurred, and you may not have found this opportunity if you hadn't jumped right on finding the solution. In the end, getting fired was the best thing that could have happened.

Example # 2

Another example would be if you are training to run a marathon and you break your ankle. You look at your other options and you decide that you will do some swimming in the meantime to keep your cardio up while you are healing. You discover that you love swimming and that you are really good at it. Then, you decide to do some swimming competitions. You would have never found out you liked this or realized you had this talent if you would have not had the challenge come up and found the solution.

You will have plenty of challenges that come up throughout your life. Recognize them. Realize that it means you are moving forward. Keep moving forward by finding the solutions to them!

It is important to be able to be a solution minded person and think up solutions on the spot, but I also think it is great to be preemptive with solution finding. So when you are working on accomplishing a new goal, it can be helpful to think of what could get in the way and how you would solve the issue. Once you have done this work do not dwell on it. It does you no good to keep thinking about what could go wrong. You only want to make sure that you have a solid foundation of what solutions can be employed for foreseen obstacle so that nothing will stop you. Let's look at what obstacles could get in the way and how you would work around them. Obviously you will have different goals and therefore different obstacles and solutions, but this will give you an idea of what you are looking for.

What obstacles could get in the way of you accomplishing your goals?
You can go as wild as you want with the "blocks". Let's take running a marathon for example:
1. I could get sick.
1. No time to train due to work.
2. Break my ankle.

Next come up with 1 or more solutions to each obstacle
1. Go walk instead of run and take tons of vitamin C and zinc.
2. Reschedule commitments, Find extra time before or after work, get someone else to cook dinner so I can use that time to train.
3. Do some weight training that does not put weight on my ankle.
4. Start swimming so I keep my cardiovascular system in shape while my ankle is healing.

What is your goal?

_____

What could get in the way of you accomplishing this goal?
Obstacles:

1._____
2._____
3._____
4._____
5._____
6._____
7._____
8._____
9._____
10._____

Next come up with 1 or more solutions to each issue
Solutions:

1._____
2._____
3._____
4._____
5._____
6._____
7._____
8._____
9._____
10._____

STEP 8- REWARDS AND CONSEQUENCES

"It is easy to dodge our responsibilities, but we cannot dodge the consequences of dodging our responsibilities" ~ Josiah Stamp

In this chapter you will write out a rewards list for sticking with your goal as well as a consequences list for not sticking with your goal. This way you will have at a glance the reasons why you should stick with the goal you have set. Print this out and hang it so you can look at it often.

These rewards and consequences should be as emotionally deep as you can possibly make them. If you tear up thinking of the reasons that you need to accomplish this goal then you are on the right track. If it feels like it's not really that big of a deal then it will not evoke any commitment from you. For me not being able to go on adventures and not being able to be active would be just about the worst thing imaginable, but for others it will be the thought of dying young and not being there for their children. This is so individual and personal. Find the emotions and reasons that get right to the core of why you chose this goal.

The list could look like this:

Consequences - The things that could happen if you do not stick to your goals (you can do more than 5)

1. I will not be able to travel like I want to, due to lack of mobility.
2. I could develop an illness like my parents.
3. I will be unable to be there for my kids the way I would like.
4. I will constantly feel self-conscious and will have a hard time finding clothing.
5. I will wind up teaching my children bad habits and set them up to have health problems.

Rewards - The good outcomes that can happen by sticking to your goals (again, you can do more than 5)

1. I will enjoy a higher quality of life with my children.
2. I will have more energy so that I enjoy my days better.
3. I will love looking in the mirror and strutting on the beach.
4. I will feel more confident and therefore my relationships will be stronger.
5. I will realize my self-worth and set more goals to accomplish things I have always wanted to.

What is your goal?

_____

Consequences

_____
_____
_____
_____
_____
_____
_____
_____
_____
_____

Rewards

_____
_____
_____
_____
_____
_____
_____
_____
_____
_____

STEP 9- TRUE IDENTITY

"In the social jungle of human existence, there is no feeling of being alive without a sense of identity" ~ *Erik Erikson*

We have words we use all the time to understand our own identity. These words can either be negative or positive, mundane or extraordinary. The thing is, what identity we *choose* for ourselves can be helpful or detrimental. That's right. You heard me. We *choose* our identity. What we say and believe plays a huge factor. By changing this, we can change how we identify ourselves.

If you are a cashier at a café, but you are working on being a professional painter, then you could choose to make your identity a painter. Sure you may still be working the cashier job, but that is not who you are. You are a painter. When someone asks you what you do you can say, "I am a painter." This does not mean that you should lie about what you do. If you tell someone you make a living as a painter but you don'tt, that is lying. That will only make you feel inconsistent. If you say that you are a film producer, but you have never done any producing, you are not taking classes or taking any steps to get closer to producing then labeling yourself as a film producer would not be consistent in your own mind because you know you are not doing anything towards it. But if it really is something that you have been doing consistently and working on, then use it!

If you are needing to make a change about a self-esteem issue, you could use "I am" statements as well. Instead of thinking that no one cares about you, replace that with "I am loveable." Along the same lines, if you are always telling yourself that you are not good at anything, change that by saying, "I am good at many things." Honestly, if you really think about it, you will find there are many things you are good at. You should think about those things you are good at when you make the "I am" statements.

Sometimes just saying "I am" is a little too intense. If you say, for instance, "I am fit" but don't believe it, then instead use, "I am becoming more fit every day." Sometimes adding that "becoming" into your "I am" statement helps you to incorporate it into your life, without the intensity it may make you feel consistent. It just can take a little of the pressure off of you if you are not feeling very confident in your statement.

We are going to go over "I am" statements on the next page, feel free to add "becoming" into your "I am" statements if it makes you feel better or more in sync with them.

The I Am's are the labels we put on ourselves. They can be both good, bad and neutral. Here are some examples of I AM:

I am a public speaker   I am a girlfriend
I am a daughter   I am old
I am healthy   I am a great communicator
I am happy   I am confident
I am lazy   I am fit

Now it's your turn!

First, list your <u>current</u> identities that you tell yourself regularly:

I AM.....

_____
_____
_____
_____
_____
_____
_____
_____

Next, think of what you want to accomplish in your life. Are you being who you need to be to accomplish your vision? Do you need to remove a negative identity or add in another positive identity that will help you to accomplish this? For instance, say you want to be the best sales person in the world, but you are lacking the confidence you need. add in, "I am confident" or "I am becoming more confident." Watch what happens.

As another example: you have been wanting to start your own business, but have not been sure about when or what you should start, or maybe you are simply unsure about yourself. Adding "I am becoming a business owner" would be a good one.

You may simply be wanting to use some "I am" statements to help you with your health and fitness level. : "I am a runner," "I am an athlete," "I am a fitness enthusiast" could all work. Everyone has different goals so everyone's "I am" statement will be different.

With that in mind, let's do another exercise!

Do you have some other identities that you could add to help you achieve your goals? If so, list them:

I AM......

Let's take this one step further.

For many, having one overall identity that you feel can encompass all of your other identities can help. It is kind of the quick reminder in your day of the power you have or who you are. It can be used as a chant in your head, or out loud when things are tough and you need some extra oomph.

For instance, mine is "I am Wonder Woman." I use this often, especially when I am working out. I will also use it when I am stressed out and need to get through a difficult time. Every time I use my chosen identity, I'm reminded that I can do anything.

I have heard people use overall identities like: "I am... an Adventurer, a superhero, a leader, lover of life, Mother, wild child, peaceful, etc." There is no right or wrong with this. It is supposed to be whatever you feel encompasses what you choose to be and what motivates to you.

What is your **one identity** that encompasses them all? Brainstorm a few, and then select the one that you like the most for yourself:

Each day repeat your positive identities out loud to yourself with conviction!

STEP 10- I DESERVE....

"You can search throughout the entire universe for someone who is more deserving of your love and affection than you are yourself, and that person is not to be found anywhere. You yourself, as much as anybody in the entire universe deserve your love and affection" ~ Buddha

Many people have a hard time believing that they really do deserve what they want for themselves. Many times these are deep-rooted beliefs, and you may need to get some professional help to deal with them. Using affirmations can be a helpful way to start boosting the belief that you deserve what you want.

"I deserve" is a great affirmation to use. When using this, say it out loud. Muster all the belief that you can about this. Think about how exciting it will be when you accomplish what you want. Put that emotion into your affirmation.

Here are some examples:
- I deserve to be fit and healthy.
- I deserve to be top in my field.
- I deserve to eat healthy food.

The point here is to start letting yourself know that you do actually deserve to have the life you want. You can create as many of these as you want. But, at the very least create one!

The lighter version.

If saying, "I deserve" is completely out of the question because you really do not feel like you deserve what you want then instead you can use, "wouldn't it be great if....." When you do this, it takes the pressure off and can help you feel the excitement of what would happen if you got what you really want, without the pressure of forcing yourself to believe it. After you do this a while, you will create more positive feelings around what you want, and then you should be able to make the leap from this lighter mode to the "I deserve" mode. That being said, if you do not believe you deserve something, you should determine whether or not this is really a goal you've set for yourself. Are you using it to please someone else instead? Is there another motivation behind it other than for yourself?

So here is your chance:

I deserve...

_____
_____
_____
_____
_____
_____
_____
_____
_____
_____
_____
_____
_____
_____
_____

Or you can use this one.

Wouldn't it be great if...

_____
_____
_____
_____
_____
_____
_____
_____
_____
_____

STEP 11 - MIND YOUR SURROUNDINGS

"We are all instruments endowed with feeling and memory. Our senses are so many strings that are struck by surrounding objects and that also frequently strike themselves." ~ Denis Diderot

Many things comprise our surroundings, and it can be either supportive or detrimental to us. Let's look at the things in our environment that influences us. We will start with the people we surround ourselves with.

You are the sum of the 6 people you spend the most time with!

Who do you hang around? Look at the people you are spending time with. Are they healthy? Do they talk about their dreams and goals? Look at their good qualities and bad qualities. Does one override the other? How do you feel when you are around them and how do you feel when you leave them?

I was dating a man whom I thought was good for me. But I felt restless when I was around him. He was not supportive of the dreams I was aiming for in my life, I love health, fitness and film. He never wanted to hear about what I was doing or read the article a magazine had written about me. In fact, instead of looking at it, he straight up told me he could not handle me doing acting ever. Rather, he wanted me to have a regular job and not take risks. All of this negativity influenced me big time because I cared about him and valued his opinion.

Another friend that I had was so much fun to be around. We always had a blast together and we spent a lot of time together. The problem was that he had a very unhealthy drinking problem so I (who had stopped drinking years earlier) started drinking with him. This lead to staying out late and not getting enough sleep and other unhealthy habits. Plus, I was acting a bit more like him. This guy told me he was an a**hole, and I blew it off as low self-esteem or joking. I will tell you that when someone says something like this, really look at it. While it might come across as joking, they may be telling you the truth. These are red flags. Take them seriously and pay close attention. Eventually, this person stabbed me in the back and that was the end of that.

On the other hand, when I lived in Texas, I had a group of friends that were amazingly supportive. We all wanted to see each other achieve our dreams. All of us had our quirky traits, and we loved that about each other. Each and every one of us wanted to do more with our lives, so we encouraged each other in those dreams. Some of us were into fitness and health, so we would go workout together. It was a great supportive environment!

I am not saying that the people you are around have to be perfect on everything because that is impossible. It is more about if they have some good qualities that you would like to emulate, and if they are supportive of who you are? I have many friends who are not into health and fitness, but they are great business people, creative artists, or just very good people in general. They all support me and cheer me on and I do the same for them. Being around people who do not support you in your dreams is draining so beware.

You are the sum of the people you spend the most time with!
Write down the top 6 people you spend the most time with on the numbered lines below. Leave the extra lines underneath the numbered ones blank for the next step:

1._____
_____
_____
_____

2._____
_____
_____
_____

3._____
_____
_____
_____

4._____
_____
_____
_____

5._____
_____
_____
_____

6._____
_____
_____
_____

Now, under each name you wrote down, list their qualities, positive and negative. This will show you the qualities you see in each person and what the balance of positive to negative is. This way you can see if maybe you would like to curtail time with them or learn how to direct the conversations with them to a more positive subject.

Your list could be that they are great at business, driven, into health, happy, lazy, negative, humble, wild, irresponsible, etc. This is for you to use. You do not need to show it to anyone else and you do not need to delete people out of your life unless you want to. So be honest. This will show you who you are spending time with so you can at least be conscious about it.

Let's look at the other aspects of these people you spend time with.

Do they support you? Do they motivate you? Or do they tell you that what you want to do is unrealistic and that you should just give it up? So many things we have in our world now were considered unrealistic when originally thought up. But that did not stop people from creating them. For instance, before they existed, a computer sounded impossible – especially one that can fit in the palm of your hand! A big hunk of metal that flies is unrealistic, but we now have airplanes. Electricity is a crazy idea and yet we have it. As Napoleon Hill said, "anything the mind can conceive and believe, it can achieve." It is true. Do not let something sounding unrealistic stop you from pursuing your dreams. After all, you may have the next big evolution for this world.

Do the people you spend time with want to see you succeed, or are they dissuading you from your path in life for "your own good"? Some friends are just helping you stay focused and some are just plain old non-supportive. The trick is recognizing which people are coming from a place of supporting you and which ones don't want you to succeed. You also may have friends that caution you if you are going to do something possibly dangerous or stupid. There is a difference between a friend being non-supportive and a friend cautioning you if you are about to step out of a plane without a parachute. No matter what anyone says, though, the choice of what you decide to do is always ultimately up to you.

What are the people you spend time with like? Do they complain or talk about possibilities? Do they take responsibility or blame others? Do they constantly say that they are in a bad situation because of their boss, how they were raised, the economy, or the weather, and there is nothing they can do about it because of someone else? Or are they the kind of people who despite what challenges are being thrown in their path, they find solutions to get through it. Do they take responsibility for their life and keep molding it into what they would like. The people you want around are those who talk about ideas and possibilities and work towards them! If *you* happen to be the person being negative you can change that! This book will help. You really can do it and have the life you want!

Now that you know the influence the people around you are having on you, start to look at who you would like to spend more time with and who you may want to spend a little less time with. Surround yourself with people that make you feel good.

Movies, Music, Books

The entertainment you partake in can have a significant effect on you as well. It is important to pay attention to how you feel when you are watching films, listening to music and reading books. If it is something that motivates you, put more of that in your life. If it is something that makes you feel bad, remove it.

Knowing how your movies, music and reading effect you is important. This way, if you are having a day where you are either feeling unmotivated or depressed you know what you can watch or read to help put you back into a good frame of mind. Different things work for different people. My movie may be Batman, Serenity or Riddick, but yours may be Zombieland or a warm and fuzzy chick flick. There is no right or wrong when it comes to what motivates you. Use whatever works for you.

I have had days when I was feeling down and just in a general funk. I would realize that I have not listened to any of my motivating music or any of my motivational books on CD in a while. Since I understand this, I can change my mood really fast. This may just be one part of motivating yourself, but every little trick we can learn helps, because you never know what is going to work for you at any given time. This will give you an idea of where to start.

What do you spend most of your time listening to and watching? Next to each write how it makes you feel (i.e. inspired, depressed, uplifted, angry, etc.):

_____

_____

_____

_____

_____

_____

_____

Which ever ones are more uplifting on this list, listen and read and watch more often. If you did not have anything on your list that makes you uplifted or motivated, then ask friends and family what works for them and check out their suggestions. If you have stuff on your list that evokes a lot of negative emotions stop watching, reading or listening to it so much!

Locations

Where we spend our time can also have a profound effect on us. The problem is it can also be so subtle that we do not realize it. Start by looking around your house. What do you have hanging in your house? Does it motivate you? What color are your walls? Is it organized the way you would like? I personally have pictures on my walls of great leaders of different industries. It reminds me to be constantly striving for more. I also have paintings I have made with motivational quotes on them and beautiful pictures. Living around motivational paintings and sayings has made a big difference for me.

Next look at your workplace. What do you have around there? Do you have wall space that you can use? If not, then where can you put things you love that you'll see every day? Can you put a personal light at your desk? That way you can have a sunlight bulb so that you can still get some of the sunny day benefits while being indoors all day? What can you add to your workplace to make it have a more positive effect on you? Most of us spend 50-60% or more of our time at our workplace, so take the time to make sure it is a place that can support you in your life instead of making it more difficult.

Find places that inspire you, where you can recharge at. I personally love the beach and the mountains. If I only have a little bit of time, maybe I will hit the beach and relax there for just a few moments to recharge. If I have a few days, I will go camping in the mountains. Between the quiet time and the beautiful surroundings, it reminds me how beautiful this world it.

How many times lately have you looked around and thought, "I love this place?" Some of us do, but many of us do not. We are going through the motions, going from work to home to work and not stopping to see what is around us. Wouldn't it be nice to go into work and actually like being there? Wouldn't it be great to go home and know that it is the custom sanctuary you created and know that you can just enjoy being there? You could look around your walls and be inspired. You can create this. It is easy, and is one simple way to subtly effect your mindset.

Does this mean that you need to immediately remodel your house to create a more motivational atmosphere? No. It means you can hang some pictures up that make you feel good. You could paint the room you spend the most time in. You could add some plants, or you could simply open some more windows to get some more light in and see the view. Again, there is no right or wrong to what you do, as long as it makes you feel more motivated, you are on the right track.

Look at what you can change at home and at work and write them below. If they seem to be a good idea, start to implement them as you can.

What changes can you make to your work space?

_____

_____

_____

_____

_____

_____

_____

_____

What changes can you make to your home?

_____

_____

_____

_____

_____

_____

_____

_____

_____

_____

_____

_____

STEP 12- DARE TO SUCK

"Take a chance! All life is a chance. The man who goes farthest is generally the one who is willing to do and dare." ~ Dale Carnegie

Many people hold themselves back from their goals because they are afraid of looking foolish. Maybe you don't want to look silly at the gym or you are afraid of doing something wrong. I have news for you. Every person who is good anything, at one point, was a beginner and had to work at it.

Everyone you see: athletes, movie stars, musicians, big business moguls and all the fitness pros were at one point just starting out. More than likely they sucked at what they were doing. Some people have a natural knack for certain things, but that does not mean that they did not have to work to get to the level they are at. Everyone starts somewhere. If you keep putting it off until you are comfortable, you will never start. Look at your favorite celebrities in any field and read their bio and what it took for them to get where they are. I can most certainly say that it was not a quick easy road, and they had many embarrassing moments.

Michael Jordan is known as one of the best players in basketball, and yet he did not start that way. He worked his butt off training harder than anyone else around him. At practices, he arrived before anyone else and left after everyone else had gone home. He had desire and drive. Even when he was told he was too short to play, he persisted and put in the effort. All of that paid off, and made him who we know him to be today. This is all because he kicked butt and dared to suck!

Madonna is a genius when it comes to keeping herself in the lime light. But she did not start off with a record contract. She spent many, many years getting to where she is now. In the beginning, she was a dancer who had to live in some pretty bad conditions while chasing her dreams. Then, she broke into the music world with a fellow dancer. She spent at least 10 years until finally getting noticed. She was even daring enough in her career to do a nude photo book! Tell me that is not a prime example of daring to suck! She was willing to risk it, which is why she made it where she is now. This doesn't mean that your risk needs to have nudity involved, but it definitely goes to show that she didn't let anything stop her. Even today, Madonna continues to risk it by testing out different mediums, such as film.

Well known are the struggles of Donald Trump. Trump is a master at taking risks and daring to suck. He has made more money than most people could ever dream of, and he has also lost more money than anyone would ever dream of. Yet, he knows this is part of the game and enjoys playing it. When he sees an opportunity or thinks of something he would like to do, he goes for it. He understands that the fun and the pay offs are in the daring to suck, and that is why he is living the lifestyle he does.

"Struggle forces us to move when we would otherwise stand still. And it leads us eventually to the full realization that success comes only through struggle. Nothing worthwhile in life is ever achieved without a struggle. If it were easy, everyone would do it. Wherever you find a successful person, you will find a person who has struggled in his or her life. Life is a struggle and the rewards go to those who meet difficulty face to face, overcome it, and move on to the next challenge." - Donald Trump

Richard Branson is the face and epitome of dare to suck, and someone I look up to. Since an early age, he has embodied this way of living. He started a magazine, a record company, and an airline. The man does anything he wants to! Along the way he had plenty of struggles to overcome as well. For one, he was dyslexic and dropped out of school at age 16. But, every day, he is constantly doing something new and daring. He understands that he will probably fail in some of the things he does, but why should that stop him? It is all about the journey. I recommend you watch his full biography. Talk about Dare to Suck!

What one thing can you do this week that would be a dare to suck risk? Write down as many idea's as you can think of, then choose one and go for it!

_____

_____

_____

_____

_____

_____

_____

_____

_____

_____

_____

_____

_____

STEP 13- YOU ARE IN CHARGE

"Anything I do, I spend a lot of time. I do it with passion and intensity. I want to be in charge" ~ Eli Broad

One of the most powerful things to realize in our lives is that we are in charge of everything! What we eat, how much money we make, how we look. We are in charge of everything in our lives. Realize that you are in charge, not your cravings, not your laziness. Say it out loud. "I AM IN CHARGE!"

When you truly believe this, you will be amazed at what you can overcome and what you can resist. This is taking responsibility for your own life. When you take responsibility for your life you will realize you can do anything you want. You simply have to want it.

Focusing on solutions comes in very handy in combination with this concept. This way you can look at your health and if it is not what you think it should be, then acknowledge that you are in charge of the health you have. You can then look for the solutions to get the health you want. But you must take action! Finding solutions and sitting on them does you no good. You must take action and create the better health you desire and deserve. **YOU ARE IN CHARGE!**

Let's take an example of a woman who goes to McDonald's all the time. We will call her Becky. Every day, Becky goes to McDonald's and orders a Big Mac, fries and a soda. Then, of course, she super sizes it. Why not, right? It's a better deal that way. The value is why Becky eats McDonalds as much as she does. It is cheap and fast. She works a lot and does not have time to cook her food. In fact, she is so busy that she has no time to workout. After a while, Becky realizes that she has gained a ton of weight and has some health issues surfacing as well. She decides that it is McDonald's fault and decides to sue them, stating that their food is bad for you and she was not warned about this.

Okay, in the situation above there are many factors. First of all, McDonald's is a restaurant. They make the food; they do not cram it down your throat. That said, Becky could have chosen better food options. Yes, even McDonald's has come up with healthier choices. She could have chosen to go to a different place for food, or found healthy frozen dinners instead. The other roads she could have chosen are endless. But here is the main factor: she did not take responsibility for her actions. Instead of being in charge of herself, she was letting other circumstances be in charge of her.

What if you are having other health situations surface that you feel are out of your control? Maybe you are dealing with fibromyalgia. Does this mean you chose to be sick? Not necessarily, but you are also not without some control. You can choose to do what you can to help the situation along. Eat a anti inflammation or candida cleansing diet. Start to workout in a way that is going to make you stronger and more in control of the pain. The point is even when you feel like you have no control, you do.

No, I am not saying that when you are starting on a healthier lifestyle that it is super easy; but, you can start with small steps and not give into your cravings 24/7. Just one healthier meal a day and a 10 minute walk can make a difference. The ultimate secret is that you have to take responsibility and be in charge of your own life. Once you are in charge, anything is possible. If you keep blaming others then you are never going to be in a position to change your life for the better. This means that having a cheeseburger or pizza is not the end of the world, but you do need to accept that it is YOUR choice. Once you take responsibility for the actions you don't like and realize that you make the choices, then you also understand that you have the power to create whatever you want with your life.

If you really are dealing with something that is out of your control, or something you just don't have any idea how to fix, you still have control over your own thoughts and emotions. You can choose to look at the situation in a different light. We always have choices even when we feel out of control.

"The question isn't who is going to let me; it's who is going to stop me." ~ Ayn Rand

YOU HAVE THE TOOLS NOW USE THEM!

I am so happy that I got to share these tools with you! Now that you have read through this book and have done the exercises in each portion, you should have a good road map to help you get on the path of what you would like to accomplish and how to accomplish them. You can use these tools as often as you like. I suggest going through them at least once a year, but it all depends on what you need. For me, I sometimes plan out my years' worth of goals and still go back through them once a month. This way, it keeps it fresh in my mind and as up-to-date as possible.

Remember to continually seek new, fresh motivation. If you start to wane in your motivation, go through this workbook again. If you are someone who needs to constantly have new motivations in your life, then I would suggest getting a few books and/or audio books that you really like and read or listen to a few pages every day. Some great books to check out are:

- <u>Unleash Your Inner Superhero</u> by Lauren Denos
- <u>Think and Grow Rich</u> by Napolean Hill
- <u>Success Principles</u> by Jack Canfield
- <u>The Slight Edge</u> by Jeff Olson
- <u>Awaken the Giant Within</u> and <u>Live with Passion</u> are just two of the great books by Tony Robbins

You can also check out my website where new health, fitness, and motivational articles go up every week. www.OneUpHealth.com

In addition to motivational and learning material I also read a lot of fictional stories to motivate me. It does not matter where you get your motivation as long as it works for you. Go ahead and put these tools to use and create the life and the health that you want. You deserve it!

ABOUT THE AUTHOR

I never thought in a million years I would be a writer. I did not believe it was my talent. But I have so much information that I want to share and want to be able to help more people, so I started. I figured this is one of the best ways to help the most people. I get better at detail and explanations with each day I write.

I started on this path because of my own health and fitness issues. At 14 I began to have others ask me questions to help them with their health, and I have been involved in health since then. It has been 21 years that I have been involved and 18 years since I have been certified in the health and fitness industry.

My desire to help others with their health and motivation came from dealing with a plethora of health issues and abuse. From an early age I dealt with allergies, gut problems, and bad body image issues, which resulted in anorexia and then weight gain. I have also dealt with blood sugar issues and other issues that would get in the way of my exercise, along with abuse at the hands of someone who supposedly loved me. This taught me a great deal, and I learned to love myself and do what is right for me. Too many of us berate ourselves for what we are not, instead of looking at what we have done with our lives and what we have in our life that is wonderful. I guarantee that you have something that is amazing about you, and are capable of doing truly wonderful things.

Through all of this I have learned to strive to always be in better health, and at the same time loving myself for who I am now. It is not about being perfect, it is about working towards being a better you. I really do believe that our health is meant to support us in our daily adventures, and when we look at it that way we will get to a good place with our health. The point is to find a better way of health that works for our individual needs and that we can live with for life, not a yo-yo diet. I also believe that life is too short and we should go after what we want in life. Staring death in the face a few times has given me the desire to really live full out. Hard times like these can either defeat us or they can grow us. We can grow to be more than we ever knew we could. I use what has happened in my life to fuel my ambition and to create a happier life. After all, life is too short not to live it.

Always *LIVE FULL OUT!*

AUTHOR CONTACT INFO

I love to hear from my community, if this book has helped you or if you have questions or comments. Feel free to email me.

Lauren Denos
Lauren@OneUpHealth.com

www.ingramcontent.com/pod-product-compliance
Lightning Source LLC
Chambersburg PA
CBHW081145290526
45795CB00006B/2380